My Vibrant Lean and Green Cooking Plan

Be Fit & Healthy with

My Ultimate Cookbook

Carmen Bellisario

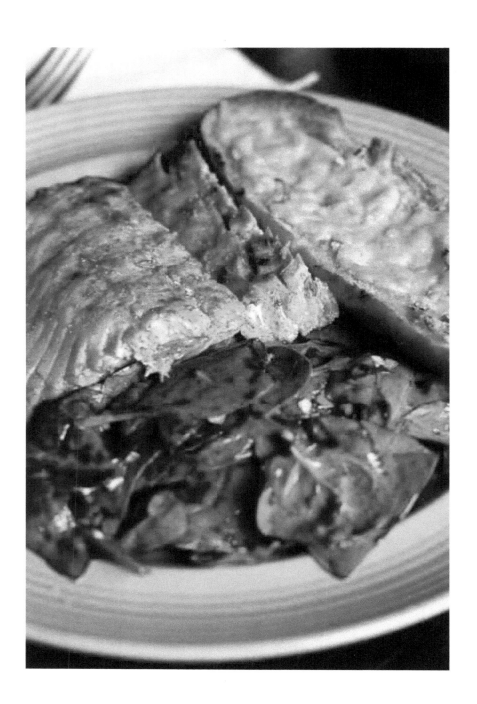

TABLE OF CONTENTS

Lemon Chili Salmon

Cooking time: 17 minutes

Servings: 4

Ingredients:

- 2 lbs. of salmon fillet; skinless and boneless
- 2 lemon juice
- 1 orange juice
- 1 tbsp. of olive oil
- 1 bunch of fresh dill
- 1 chili; sliced
- Pepper
- Salt

Directions:

1. Preheat the air fryer to 3250 F.
2. Place salmon fillets in air fryer baking pan and drizzle with olive oil, lime juice, and orange juice.
3. Sprinkle chili slices over salmon and season with pepper and salt.
4. Place pan in the air fryer and cook for 15-17 minutes.

5. Garnish with dill and serve.

Nutrition:

- Calories: 339
- Fat: 17.5 g
- Carbohydrates: 2 g
- Sugar: 2 g
- Protein: 44 g
- Cholesterol: 100 mg

Cajun Seasoned Salmon Filet

Preparation time: 5 minutes

Cooking time: 15 minutes

Servings: 1

Ingredients:

- 1 salmon fillet
- 1 teaspoon of juice from lemon; freshly squeezed
- 3 tablespoons of extra virgin olive oil
- A dash of Cajun seasoning mix

Directions:

1. Preheat the air fryer for 5 minutes.
2. Place all Ingredients in a bowl and toss to coat.
3. Place the fillet in the air fryer basket.
4. Bake for 15 minutes at 3250 F. Once cooked, drizzle with olive oil.

Nutrition:

- Calories: 523

- Carbohydrates: 4.6 g
- Protein: 47.9 g
- Fat: 34.8 g

Apple Slaw Topped Alaskan Cod Filet

Preparation time: 5 minutes

Cooking time: 15 minutes

Servings: 3

Ingredients:

- ¼ cup of mayonnaise
- ½ red onion; diced
- 1 ½ pounds of frozen Alaskan cod
- 1 box of whole wheat panko bread crumbs
- 1 granny smith apple; julienned
- 1 tablespoon of vegetable oil
- 1 teaspoon of paprika
- 2 cups of Napa cabbage; shredded
- Salt and pepper to taste

Directions:

1. Preheat the air fryer to 3900 F.
2. Place the grill pan accessory in the air fryer.

3. Brush the fish with oil and dredge in the breadcrumbs.
4. Place the fish on the grill pan and cook for 15 minutes. Make sure to flip the fish halfway through the Cooking time.
5. Meanwhile, prepare the slaw by mixing the remaining Ingredients in a bowl.
6. Serve the fish with the slaw.

Nutrition:

- Calories: 316
- Carbs: 13.5g
- Protein: 37.8g
- Fat: 12.2g

Pesto Salmon

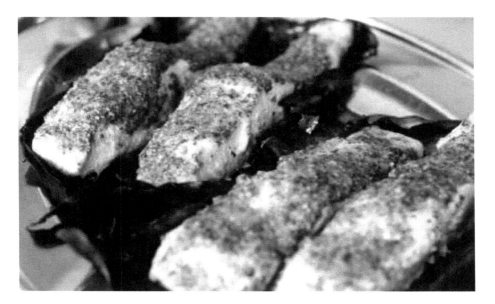

Cooking time: 16 minutes

Servings: 4

Ingredients:

- 25 oz. of salmon fillet
- 1 tbsp. of green pesto
- 1 cup of mayonnaise
- 1/2 oz. of olive oil
- 1 lb. of fresh spinach
- 2 oz. of parmesan cheese; grated
- Pepper
- Salt

Directions:

1. Preheat the air fryer to 3700 F.
2. Spray air fryer basket with cooking spray.
3. Season salmon fillet with pepper and salt and place into the air fryer basket.
4. In a bowl, mix together the mayonnaise, parmesan cheese, pesto, and cover the salmon fillet.
5. Cook salmon for 14-16 minutes.
6. Meanwhile, in a pan sauté spinach with olive oil until spinach is wilted, or for about 2-3 minutes. Season with pepper and salt.
7. Transfer spinach to serving plate and top with cooked salmon.
8. Serve and enjoy.

Nutrition:

- Calories: 545
- Fat: 39.6 g
- Carbohydrates: 9.5 g
- Sugar: 3.1 g
- Protein: 43 g
- Cholesterol: 110 mg

Parmesan Walnut Salmon

Preparation time: 10 minutes

Cooking time: 12 minutes

Servings: 4

Ingredients:

- 4 salmon fillets
- 1/4 cup of parmesan cheese; grated
- 1/2 cup of walnuts
- 1 tsp. of olive oil
- 1 tbsp. of lemon rind

Directions:

1. Preheat the air fryer to 3700 F.
2. Spray an air fryer baking dish with cooking spray.
3. Place salmon on a baking dish.
4. Add walnuts into the food processor and process until finely ground.
5. Mix ground walnuts with parmesan cheese, olive oil, and lemon peel. Stir well.
6. Spoon walnut mixture over the salmon and press gently.

7. Place in the air fryer and cook for 12 minutes.

8. Serve and enjoy.

Nutrition:

- Calories: 420
- Fat: 27.4 g
- Carbohydrates: 2 g
- Sugar: 0.3 g
- Protein: 46.3 g
- Cholesterol: 98 mg

Air Fried Cod with Basil Vinaigrette

Preparation time: 5 minutes

Cooking time: 15 minutes

Servings: 4

Ingredients:

- ¼ cup o olive oil
- 4 cod fillets
- A bunch of basil; torn
- Juice from 1 lemon; freshly squeezed
- Salt and pepper to taste

Directions:

1. Preheat the air fryer for 5 minutes.
2. Season the cod fillets with salt and pepper to taste.
3. Place in the air fryer and cook for 15 minutes at 350 0 F.
4. Meanwhile, put the rest of the Ingredients in a bowl and toss to mix.
5. Serve the air fried cod with the basil vinaigrette.

Nutrition:

- Calories: 235
- Carbohydrates: 1.9 g
- Protein: 14.3 g
- Fat: 18.9 g

Lemon Shrimp

Preparation time: 10 minutes

Cooking time: 8 minutes

Servings: 2

Ingredients:

- 12 oz. of shrimp; peeled and deveined
- 1 lemon; sliced
- 1/4 tsp. of garlic powder
- 1/4 tsp. of paprika
- 1 tsp. of lemon pepper
- 1 lemon juice
- 1 tbsp. of olive oil

Directions:

1. In a bowl, mix together the oil, lemon juice, garlic powder, paprika, and lemon pepper.
2. Add shrimp to the bowl and toss well to coat.
3. Spray air fryer basket with cooking spray.
4. Transfer shrimp into the air fryer basket and cook at 4000 F for 8 minutes.

5. Garnish with lemon slices and serve.

Nutrition:

- Calories: 381
- Fat: 17.1 g
- Carbohydrates: 4.1 g
- Sugar: 0.6 g
- Protein: 50.6 g
- Cholesterol: 358 mg

Filipino Bistek

Preparation time: 5 minutes

Cooking time: 10 minutes

Servings: 4

Ingredients:

- 2 milkfish bellies; deboned and sliced into 4 portions
- ¾ tsp. of salt
- ¼ tsp. of ground black pepper
- ¼ tsp. of cumin powder
- 2 tbsps. of calamansi juice
- 2 lemongrasses; trimmed and cut crosswise into small pieces
- ½ cup of tamari sauce
- 2 tbsps. of fish sauce
- 2 tbsps. of sugar
- 1 tsp. of garlic powder
- ½ cup of chicken broth
- 2 tbsps. of olive oil

Directions:

1. Dry the fish using some paper towels.
2. Put the fish in a large bowl and coat with the rest of the Ingredients. Allow to chill for 3 hours in the refrigerator.
3. Cook the fish steaks on an Air Fryer grill basket at 340°F for 5 minutes.
4. Turn the steaks over and allow to grill for a further 4 minutes. Cook until light brown.
5. Serve with steamed polished rice.

Nutrition:

- Calories: 259
- Fat: 3 g
- Protein: 10 g
- Sugar: 2 g

Saltine Fish Fillets

Preparation time: 10 minutes

Cooking time: 15 minutes

Servings: 4

Ingredients:

- 1 cup of crushed saltines
- ¼ cup of extra-virgin olive oil
- 1 tsp. of garlic powder
- ½ tsp. of shallot powder
- 1 egg; well whisked
- 4 white fish fillets
- Salt and ground black pepper to taste
- Fresh Italian parsley to serve

Directions:

1. In a shallow bowl, mix the crushed saltines and olive oil.
2. In a separate bowl, mix together the garlic powder, shallot powder, and the beaten egg.
3. Sprinkle a good amount of salt and pepper over the fish, before dipping each fillet into the egg mixture.

4. Coat the fillets with the crumb mixture.

5. Air fry the fish at 370°F for 10-12 minutes.

6. Serve with fresh parsley.

Nutrition:

- Calories: 502
- Fat: 4 g
- Protein: 11 g
- Sugar: 9 g

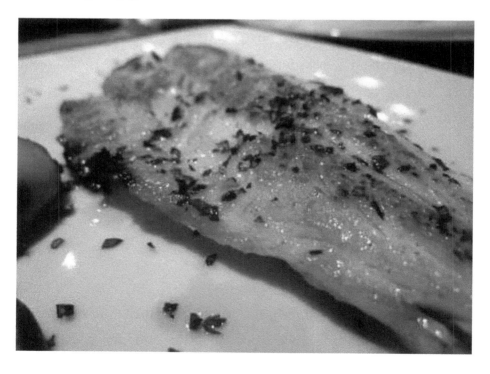

Another Crispy Coconut Shrimp Recipe

Preparation time: 5 minutes

Cooking time: 20 minutes

Servings: 4

Ingredients:

- ½ cup of flour
- ½ stick of cold butter; cut into cubes
- ½ tablespoon of lemon juice
- 1 egg yolk; beaten
- 1 green onion; chopped
- 1-pound of salmon fillets; cut into small cubes
- 3 tablespoons of whipping cream
- 4 eggs; beaten
- Salt and pepper to taste

Directions:

1. Preheat the air fryer to 3900 F.
2. Season salmon fillets with lemon juice, salt, and pepper.

3. In another bowl, mix the flour and butter. Add cold water gradually to make a dough. Knead the dough on a flat surface to make a sheet.
4. Place the dough on the baking dish and press firmly on the dish.
5. Beat the eggs and Ingredients and season with salt and pepper to taste.
6. Place the salmon cubes on the pan lined with dough and pour the egg over.
7. Cook for 15 to 20 minutes.
8. Garnish with green onions once cooked.

Nutrition:

- Calories: 483
- Carbs: 5.2 g
- Protein: 45.2 g
- Fat: 31.2 g

Baked Scallops with Garlic Aioli

Preparation time: 5 minutes

Cooking time: 10 minutes

Servings: 4

Ingredients:

- 1 cup of bread crumbs
- 1/4 cup of chopped parsley
- 16 sea scallops; rinsed and drained
- 2 shallots; chopped
- 3 pinches of ground nutmeg
- 4 tablespoons of olive oil
- 5 cloves garlic; minced
- 5 tablespoons of butter; melted
- Salt and pepper to taste

Directions:

1. Lightly grease baking pan of air fryer with cooking spray.
2. Mix in shallots, garlic, melted butter, and scallops. Season with pepper, salt, and nutmeg.

3. In a small bowl, whisk well the olive oil and bread crumbs. Sprinkle over scallops.
4. Cook on 3900 F for 10 minutes, or until tops are lightly brown.
5. Serve and enjoy with a sprinkle of parsley.

Nutrition:

- Calories 452
- Carbs: 29.8 g
- Protein: 15.2 g
- Fat: 30.2 g

Basil 'n Lime-Chili Clams

Preparation time: 5 minutes

Cooking time: 15 minutes

Servings: 3

Ingredients:

- ½ cup of basil leaves
- ½ cup of tomatoes; chopped
- 1 tablespoon of fresh lime juice
- 25 littleneck clams
- 4 cloves of garlic; minced
- 6 tablespoons of unsalted butter
- Salt and pepper to taste

Directions:

1. Preheat the air fryer to 3900 F.
2. Place the grill pan accessory in the air fryer.
3. Place all Ingredients on a large foil. Fold over the foil and close by crimping the edges.
4. Place on the grill pan and cook for 15 minutes.
5. Serve with bread.

Nutrition:

- Calories: 163
- Carbs: 4.1 g
- Protein: 1.7 g
- Fat: 15.5 g

Beer Battered Cod Filet

Preparation time: 5 minutes

Cooking time: 15 minutes

Servings: 2

Ingredients:

- ½ cup of all-purpose flour
- ¾ teaspoon of baking powder
- 1 ¼ cup of lager beer
- 2 cod fillets
- 2 eggs; beaten
- Salt and pepper to taste

Directions:

1. Preheat the air fryer to 3900 F.
2. Pat the fish fillets dry then put aside.
3. In a bowl, mix the rest of the Ingredients to make a batter.
4. Dip the fillets in the batter and place on the double layer rack.
5. Cook for 15 minutes.

Nutrition:

- Calories: 229
- Carbs: 33.2 g
- Protein: 31.1 g
- Fat: 10.2 g

Butterflied Prawns with Garlic-Sriracha

Preparation time: 5 minutes

Cooking time: 15 minutes

Servings: 2

Ingredients:

- 1 tablespoon of lime juice
- 1 tablespoon of sriracha
- 1-pound of large prawns; shells removed and cut lengthwise or butterflied
- 1teaspoon of fish sauce
- 2 tablespoons of melted butter
- 2 tablespoons of minced garlic
- Salt and pepper to taste

Directions:

1. Preheat the air fryer to 3900 F.
2. Place the grill pan accessory in the air fryer.
3. Season the prawns with the rest of the Ingredients.

4. Place on the grill pan and cook for 15 minutes. Make sure you flip the prawns halfway through the Cooking time.

Nutrition:

- Calories: 443
- Carbs: 9.7 g
- Protein: 62.8 g
- Fat: 16.9 g

Bass Filet in Coconut Sauce

Preparation time: 5 minutes

Cooking time: 15 minutes

Servings: 4

Ingredients:

- ¼ cup of coconut milk
- ½ pound of bass fillet
- 1 tablespoon of olive oil
- 2 tablespoons of jalapeno; chopped
- 2 tablespoons of lime juice; freshly squeezed
- 3 tablespoons of parsley; chopped
- Salt and pepper to taste

Directions:

1. Preheat the air fryer for 5 minutes
2. Season the bass with salt and pepper to taste. Brush the surface with olive oil.
3. Place in the air fryer and cook for 15 minutes at 3500 F.
4. Meanwhile, place in a saucepan the coconut milk, lime juice, jalapeno, and parsley.

5. Heat over medium flame.
6. Serve the fish with the coconut sauce.

Nutrition:

- Calories: 139
- Carbohydrates: 2.7 g
- Protein: 8.7 g
- Fat: 10.3 g

Arugula and Sweet Potato Salad

Preparation time: 10 minutes

Cooking time: 20 minutes

Servings: 4

Ingredients:

- 1 lb. of sweet potatoes
- 1 cup of walnuts
- 1 tablespoon of olive oil
- 1 cup of water
- 1 tablespoon of soy sauce
- 3 cups of arugula

Directions:

1. Bake potatoes at 4000 F until they are soft, then remove and put aside.
2. In a bowl, drizzle walnuts with olive oil and microwave for 2-3 minutes or until toasted.
3. In a bowl, combine all salad Ingredients and blend well.
4. Pour over soy and serve.

Nutrition:

- Calories: 189
- Total Carbohydrate: 2 g
- Cholesterol: 13 mg
- Total Fat: 7 g
- Fiber: 2 g
- Protein: 10 g
- Sodium: 301 mg

Nicoise Salad

Preparation time: 15 minutes

Cooking time: 10 minutes

Servings: 4

Ingredients:

- 1 oz. of red potatoes
- 1 package of green beans
- 2 eggs
- ½ cup of tomatoes
- 2 tablespoons of wine vinegar
- ¼ teaspoon of salt
- ½ teaspoon of pepper
- ½ teaspoon of thyme
- ¼ cup of olive oil
- 6 oz. of tuna
- ¼ cup of Kalamata olives

Directions:

1. In a bowl, mix all the Ingredients together.
2. Add salad dressing and serve.

Nutrition:

- Calories: 189
- Total Carbohydrate: 2 g
- Cholesterol: 13 mg
- Total Fat: 7 g
- Fiber: 2 g
- Protein: 15 g
- Sodium: 321 mg

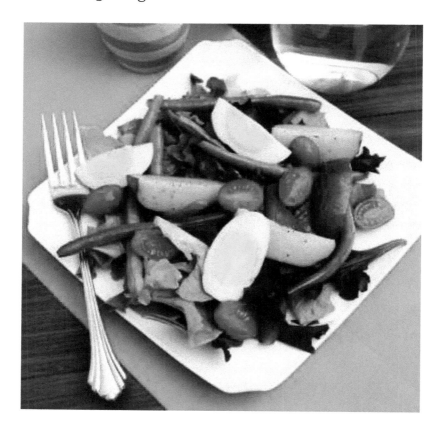

Scrambled Eggs with Goat Cheese and Roasted Peppers

Preparation time: 5 minutes

Cooking time: 10 minutes

Servings: 4

Ingredients:

- 1 1/2 teaspoons of extra-virgin olive oil
- 1 cup of chopped bell peppers; any color (about 1 medium pepper)
- 2 garlic cloves; minced (about 1 teaspoon)
- 6 large eggs
- 1/4 teaspoon of kosher or sea salt
- 2 tablespoons of water
- 1/2 cup of crumbled goat cheese (about 2 ounces)
- 2 tablespoons of loosely packed chopped fresh mint

Directions:

1. In a large skillet, heat the oil over medium-high heat. Add the peppers and cook for 5 minutes, stirring occasionally.

2. Add the garlic and cook for 1 minute.
3. While the peppers are cooking, whisk together the eggs, salt, and water in a medium bowl.
4. Turn the heat right down to medium-low.
5. Pour the egg mixture over the peppers.
6. Let the eggs cook undisturbed for 1 to 2 minutes, or until they start to set on the bottom.
7. Sprinkle with the chevre.
8. Cook the eggs for about 1 to 2 more minutes, stirring slowly, until the eggs are soft-set and custardy.
9. Top with the fresh mint and serve.

Nutrition:

- Calories: 201
- Fat: 15 g
- Cholesterol: 294 mg
- Sodium: 176 mg
- Carbohydrates: 5 g
- Fiber: 2 g
- Protein: 15 g

Marinara Eggs with Parsley

Preparation time: 5 minutes

Cooking time: 15 minutes

Servings: 6

Ingredients:

- 1 tablespoon of extra-virgin olive oil
- 1 cup of chopped onion (about 1/2 medium onion)
- 2 garlic cloves; minced (about 1 teaspoon)
- 2 (14.5-ounce) cans of Italian diced tomatoes; undrained, no salt added
- 6 large eggs
- 1/2 cup of chopped fresh flat-leaf (Italian) parsley
- Crusty Italian bread and grated Parmesan or Romano cheese, for serving (optional)

Directions:

1. In a large skillet, heat the oil over medium-high heat.
2. Add the onion and cook for 5 minutes, stirring occasionally.
3. Add the garlic and cook for 1 minute.
4. Pour the tomatoes with their juices over the onion mixture and cook until it is bubbling, or for 2 to 3 minutes.

5. While waiting for the tomato mixture to bubble, crack one egg into a little custard cup or mug.

6. When the tomato mixture bubbles, lower the heat to medium.

7. Then use a large spoon to form 6 indentations in the tomato mixture.

8. Gently pour the first cracked egg into one indentation and repeat, cracking the remaining eggs, one at a time, into the custard cup and pouring one into each indentation.

9. Cover the skillet and cook for 6 to 7 minutes, or until the eggs are done to your liking (about 6 minutes for soft cooked, 7 minutes for harder cooked).

10. Top with the parsley, and serve with the bread and cheese, if desired.

Nutrition:

- Calories: 122
- Fat: 7 g
- Cholesterol: 186 mg
- Sodium: 207 mg
- Carbohydrates: 7 g
- Fiber: 1 g
- Protein: 7 g

Buffalo Chicken Strips

Preparation time: 5 minutes

Cooking time: 25 minutes

Servings: 1

Ingredients:

- ¼ cup of hot sauce
- 1 lb. of boneless skinless chicken tenders
- 1 tsp. of garlic powder
- 1 ½ oz. of pork rinds; finely ground
- 1 tsp. of chili powder

Directions:

1. Toss the sauce and chicken tenders together in a bowl, ensuring the chicken is totally coated.
2. In another bowl, mix the garlic powder, ground pork rinds, and chili powder. Use this mixture to coat the tenders, covering them well. Place the chicken in your fryer, taking care not to layer pieces on top of one another.

3. Cook the chicken at 375°F for 20 minutes or until cooked all the way through and golden. Serve warm together with your favorite dips and sides.

Nutrition:

- Calories: 143
- Fat: 29 g
- Carbs: 15 g
- Protein: 30 g

Quinoa-Kale Egg Casserole

Preparation time: 20 minutes

Cooking time: 6 to 8 hours

Servings: 8

Ingredients:

- 11/2 cups of roasted vegetable broth
- 11 eggs
- 11/2 cups of quinoa; rinsed and drained
- 3 cups of chopped kale
- 1 leek; chopped
- 1 red bell pepper; stemmed, seeded, and chopped
- 3 garlic cloves; minced
- 1 1/2 cups of shredded Havarti cheese

Directions:

1. Grease a 6-quart slow cooker with oil and put aside.
2. In a large bowl, mix the milk, vegetable broth, eggs, and beat well with a wire whisk.
3. Stir in the quinoa, kale, leek, bell pepper, garlic, and cheese. Pour this mixture into the prepared slow cooker.

4. Cover and cook on low for 6 to 8 hours, or until a food thermometer registers 165°F and the mixture is settled.

Nutrition:

- Calories: 483 Cal
- Carbohydrates: 32 g
- Sugar: 8 g
- Fiber: 3 g
- Fat: 27 g
- Saturated Fat: 14 g
- Protein: 25 g
- Sodium: 462 mg

Chicken and Pasta Casserole

Preparation time: 15 minutes

Cooking time: 20 minutes

Servings: 6

Ingredients:

- 8 ounces of dry fusilli pasta
- 1 1/2 ounces of olive oil
- 6 chicken tenderloins, cut in bite-sized chunks
- 1 tablespoon of dried minced onion
- A pinch of salt and pepper
- A bit of garlic powder
- ½ ounce of basil; dried
- ½ ounce of parsley; dried
- 10 3/4 ounces of condensed cream of chicken soup
- 10 3/4 ounces of condensed cream of mushroom soup
- 16 ounces of frozen mixed vegetables
- 8 ounces of bread crumbs
- 1-ounce of Parmesan cheese; grated
- 1-ounce of melted butter

Directions:

1. Preheat oven to 4000 F.
2. Lightly coat a baking dish with cooking spray.
3. Boil a large pot of salted water and cook fusilli noodles in it for 10 minutes or until tender but firm to the bite.
4. Drain water out of the pot.
5. Heat oil in a large frying pan on medium heat. Cook chicken in the oil with onion, salt, pepper, garlic powder, basil, and parsley for 20 minutes or until juices run clear.
6. Stir in pasta, soups, and vegetables. Pour the mixture into the baking dish.
7. Mix bread crumbs, parmesan and butter in a small bowl and cover the pasta.
8. Bake for 20 minutes or until browned and bubbly.

Nutrition:

- Calories: 416 Cal
- Carbohydrates: 33 g
- Sugar: 18 g
- Fiber: 15 g

Egg Mushroom Omelet

Preparation time: 5 minutes

Cooking time: 5 minutes

Servings: 2

Ingredients:

- 3 eggs
- 1 cup of button mushroom; chopped
- 1 baby shallot; chopped
- Sea salt to taste
- Cayenne pepper to taste
- 1 tbsp. of olive oil

Directions:

1. In a bowl, beat the eggs with sea salt and cayenne pepper.
2. Heat the oil in a skillet over medium heat.
3. Pour in the egg mixture.
4. Cook for 1 minute and add the mushroom and shallots.
5. Cover and cook for 2 minutes.
6. Allow to cool and serve.

Nutrition:

- Fat: 75 g
- Protein: 18 g
- Sodium: 195 mg

Egg Avocado Toast

Preparation time: 5 minutes

Cooking time: 5 minutes

Servings: 2

Ingredients:

- 2 almond bread slices
- 2 eggs
- 1 cup of avocado puree
- Sea salt to taste
- 1 tbsp. of almond butter
- Cayenne pepper to taste
- 1 tsp. of chives; chopped

Directions:

1. Toast the bread slices.
2. Spread the avocado puree onto the bread slices.
3. In a pan, add the almond butter and melt over medium heat.
4. Add the eggs and whisk for 1 minute.
5. Add the salt and cayenne pepper.

6. Scramble for 1 minute and add on top of the toast.

7. Add the chives, more salt, and pepper on top.

Nutrition:

- Fat: 18.2 g
- Carbohydrates: 19.3 g
- Fiber: 9.8 g
- Protein: 14.6 g
- Sugar: 2.9 g
- Sodium: 252 mg

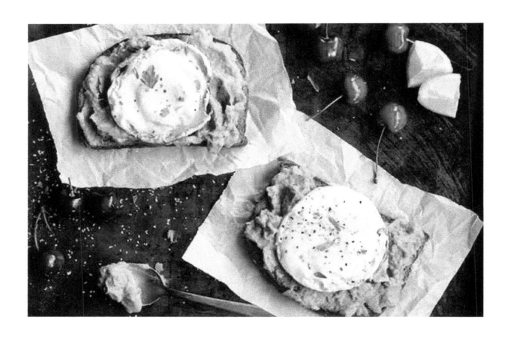

Buffalo Chicken Tenders

Preparation time: 12 minutes

Cooking time: 8 minutes

Servings: 4

Ingredients:

- 1 egg
- 1 cup of mozzarella cheese; shredded
- ¼ cup of buffalo sauce
- 1 cup of cooked chicken; shredded
- ¼ cup of feta cheese

Directions:

1. Mix all the Ingredients (except for the feta). Line the basket of your fryer with a suitably sized piece of parchment paper. Lay the mixture into the fryer and press it into a circle about half inch thick. Crumble the feta cheese over it.
2. Cook for 8 minutes at 400°F. Turn the fryer off and allow the chicken to rest inside before removing with care.
3. Cut the mixture into slices and serve hot.

Nutrition:

- Calories: 240
- Fat: 10g
- Carbs: 20 g
- Protein: 20 g

Homemade Chicken Broth

Preparation time: 5 minutes

Cooking time: 30 minutes

Servings: 4

Ingredients:

- 1 tablespoon of olive oil
- 1 chopped onion
- 2 chopped stalks celery
- 2 chopped carrots
- 1 whole chicken
- 2+ quarts of water
- 1 tablespoon of salt
- ½ teaspoon of pepper
- 1 teaspoon of fresh sage

Directions:

1. Sauté vegetables in oil.
2. Mix chicken and water and simmer for 2+ hours or until the chicken falls off the bone. Keep adding water as required.

3. Remove the chicken meat from the broth, place on a platter, and let it cool. Pull chicken off the carcass and put it into the broth.
4. Pour broth mixture into pint and quart mason jars. Make sure to add meat to every jar.
5. Leave one full inch of space from the top of the jar or it will crack when it freezes and liquids expand. Jars can stay in freezer for up to a year.
6. Take out and use whenever you make a soup.

Nutrition:

- Calories: 213
- Fat: 6 g
- Fiber: 13 g
- Carbs: 16 g
- Protein: 22 g

Fish Stew

Preparation time: 5 minutes

Cooking time: 30 minutes

Servings: 4

Ingredients:

- 1 tablespoon of olive oil
- 1 chopped onion or leek
- 2 chopped stalks celery
- 2 chopped carrots
- 1 clove of minced garlic
- 1 tablespoon of parsley
- 1 bay leaf
- 1 clove
- 1/8 teaspoon of kelp or dulse (seaweed)
- ¼ teaspoon of salt
- Fish—leftover, cooked, diced
- 2–3 cups of chicken or vegetable broth

Directions:

1. Mix all of the Ingredients and simmer on the stove for 20 minutes.

Nutrition:

- Calories: 342
- Fat: 15 g
- Fiber: 11 g
- Carbs: 8 g
- Protein: 10 g

Roasted Tomato and Seafood Stew

Preparation time: 10 minutes

Cooking time: 46 minutes

Servings: 6

Ingredients:

- 2 tablespoons of extra-virgin olive oil
- 1 yellow onion; diced
- 1 fennel bulb; tops removed and bulb diced
- 3 garlic cloves; minced
- 1 cup of dry white wine
- 2 (14.5-ounce) cans of fire-roasted tomatoes
- 2 cups of chicken stock
- 1-pound of medium (21-30 count) shrimp; peeled and deveined
- 1-pound of raw white fish (cod or haddock); cubed
- Salt
- Freshly ground black pepper
- Fresh basil; torn, for garnish

Directions:

1. Select roast/sauté and set to med. Press start/stop to start. Allow to preheat for 3 minutes.
2. Add the olive oil, onions, fennel, and garlic. Cook for about 3 minutes, or until translucent.
3. Add the wine and deglaze, scraping any stuck bits from the bottom of the pot using a silicone spatula. Add the roasted tomatoes and chicken broth. Simmer for 25 to 30 minutes. Add the shrimp and white fish.
4. Select roast/sauté and set to medium-low. Press start/stop to start.
5. Simmer for 10 minutes, stirring frequently, until the shrimp and fish are cooked through. Season with salt and pepper.
6. Ladle into bowl and serve topped with torn basil.

Nutrition:

- Calories: 301
- Total fat: 8 g
- Saturated Fat: 1 g
- Cholesterol: 99 mg
- Sodium: 808 mg
- Carbohydrates: 21 g
- Fiber: 4 g
- Protein: 26 g

White Bean and Cabbage Soup

Preparation time: 5 minutes

Cooking time: 30 minutes

Servings: 4

Ingredients:

- 1 tablespoon of olive oil
- 4 chopped carrots
- 4 chopped stalks of celery or 1 chopped bok choy
- 1 chopped onion
- 2 cloves of minced garlic
- 1 chopped cabbage head
- ½ lb. of northern beans soaked in water overnight (drained)
- 6 cups of chicken broth
- 3 cups of water

Directions:

1. Sauté vegetables in oil.
2. Add the rest of the Ingredients and cook on medium-low heat for 30 minutes.

Nutrition:

- Calories: 423
- Fat: 2 g
- Fiber: 0 g
- Carbs: 20 g
- Protein: 33 g

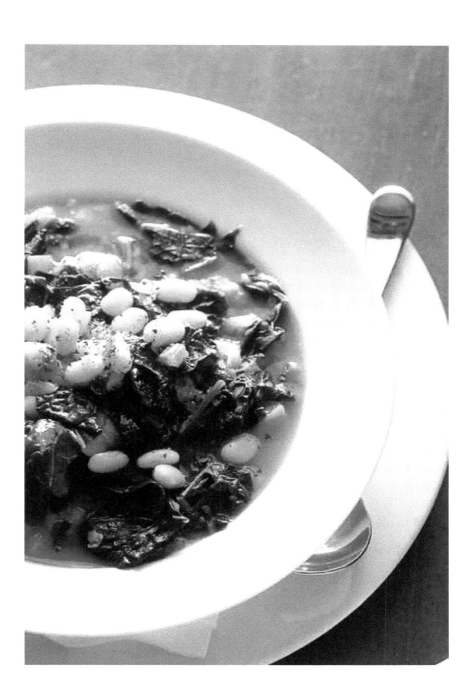

Brooke's Chili

Cooking time: 1 hour

Servings: 4

Ingredients:

- 2 lb. of organic ground beef
- 1 diced onion
- 3 cloves of minced garlic
- 6 diced tomatoes
- 1 jar of tomato sauce
- 1 tablespoon of salt
- 1 cup of water
- 1 cup of kidney beans soaked in water overnight (drained)
- 1 cup of pinto beans soaked in water overnight (drained)
- 2 tablespoons of chili powder
- 1 tablespoon of cumin
- 1 tablespoon of honey or maple syrup
- 1 teaspoon of baking stevia
- 1 teaspoon of pepper

Directions:

1. In a large pot, brown the ground beef and drain the oil.
2. Add the onion and garlic and cook until translucent.
3. Add the rest of the Ingredients and simmer for 1 hour.

Nutrition:

- Calories: 110
- Fat: 31 g
- Fiber: 18 g
- Carbs: 15 g
- Protein: 12 g

Flavorful Broccoli Soup

Preparation time: 10 minutes

Cooking time: 4 hours 15 minutes

Servings: 6

Ingredients:

- 20 oz. of broccoli florets
- 4 oz. of cream cheese
- 8 oz. of cheddar cheese; shredded
- 1/2 tsp. of paprika
- 1/2 tsp. of ground mustard
- 3 cups of chicken stock
- 2 garlic cloves; chopped
- 1 onion; diced
- 1 cup of carrots; shredded
- 1/4 tsp. of baking soda
- 1/4 tsp. of salt

Directions:

1. Add all the Ingredients except cream cheese and cheddar cheese to a Crock Pot and stir well.

2. Cover and cook on low for 4 hours.
3. Purée the soup using an immersion blender until it's smooth.
4. Stir in the cream cheese and cheddar cheese.
5. Cover and cook on low for 15 minutes more.
6. Season with pepper and salt.
7. Serve and enjoy.

Nutrition:

- Calories 275
- Fat 19 g
- Carbohydrates 19 g
- Sugar 4 g
- Protein 14 g
- Cholesterol 60 mg

Lentil Soup

Cooking time: 2 hours

Servings: 4

Ingredients:

- 2 tablespoons of olive oil
- 2 chopped onions
- 1 chopped red pepper
- 1 chopped carrot
- 2 cloves of minced garlic
- ½ teaspoon of cumin
- ¾ teaspoon of thyme
- 1 bay leaf
- 8 cups of chicken broth
- 2 chopped tomatoes
- ½ pound of dried lentils (1¼ cup)
- Optional: add bacon or ham to flavor.
- 1 teaspoon of salt
- ¼ teaspoon of pepper
- Handful of spinach

Directions:

1. Sauté vegetables in oil.
2. Mix all the Ingredients (except spinach and spices).
3. Cover and cook on low for 2 hours.
4. Add spinach and spices.

Nutrition:

- Calories: 257
- Fat: 13 g
- Fiber: 37 g
- Carbs: 11g
- Protein: 8 g

White Chicken Chili

Cooking time: 30 minutes

Servings: 4

Ingredients:

- 1 tablespoon of olive oil
- 1 pound of chicken strips cut into pieces
- 2 teaspoons of cumin
- ½ teaspoon of oregano
- ½ teaspoon of salt
- ½ teaspoon of pepper
- 1 chopped onion
- 1 chopped red bell pepper
- 4 cloves of minced garlic
- 4 cups of chicken broth
- 2 cups of northern beans soaked in water overnight (drained)

Directions:

1. Sauté chicken and spices in oil and remove from pan.
2. Sauté onion and red pepper.

3. Add all of the Ingredients including chicken into a pot and cook on medium-low heat for 15 minutes.

Nutrition:

- Calories: 208
- Fat: 3 g
- Fiber: 4 g
- Carbs: 7 g
- Protein: 27 g

Black Bean Soup

Preparation time: 5 minutes

Cooking time: 1 hour

Servings: 4

Ingredients:

- 1 pound of dry black beans (soak in water overnight and drain water)
- 1 tablespoon of olive oil
- 2 cups of chopped onion or 1 leek
- 1 cup of chopped carrots
- 4 cloves of minced garlic
- 2 teaspoons of cumin
- ¼ teaspoon of red pepper flakes
- 4 cups of chicken broth
- 4 cups of water
- ¼ teaspoon of thyme
- 2 chopped tomatoes or 1 (14 oz.) can tomatoes
- 1½ teaspoon of salt
- Optional: add bacon or ham to flavor.
- Chopped green onions to garnish

Directions:

1. Sauté vegetables in oil. Add all of the Ingredients and cook on stovetop on medium-low heat for 1 hour.

Nutrition:

- Calories: 508
- Fat: 12 g
- Fiber: 9 g
- Carbs: 24 g
- Protein: 40 g

Homemade Vegetable Broth

Preparation time: 5 minutes

Cooking time: 30 minutes

Servings: 4

Ingredients:

- 1 tablespoon of olive oil
- 1 chopped onion
- 2 chopped stalks celery
- 2 chopped carrots
- 1 head of bok choy
- 6 cups or 1 package fresh spinach
- 2+ quarts of water
- 1 tablespoon of salt
- ½ teaspoon of pepper
- 1 teaspoon fresh sage

Directions:

1. Sauté vegetables in oil. Add water and simmer for 1 hour.
2. Keep adding water as required.
3. Pour broth mixture into pint and quart mason jars.

4. Leave one full inch of space from the top of the jar or it will crack when it freezes and liquid expand. Jars can stay in freezer for up to a year.

5. Take out and use whenever you make a soup.

Nutrition:

- Calories: 140
- Fat: 2 g
- Fiber: 23 g
- Carbs: 22 g
- Protein: 47 g

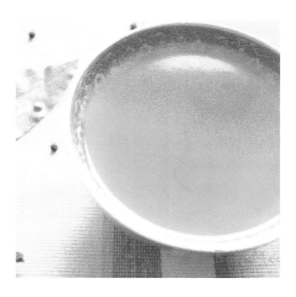

Tasty Basil Tomato Soup

Preparation time: 10 minutes

Cooking time: 6 hours

Servings: 6

Ingredients:

- 28 oz. of can whole peeled tomatoes
- 1/2 cup of fresh basil leaves
- 4 cups of chicken stock
- 1 tsp. of red pepper flakes
- 3 garlic cloves; peeled
- 2 onions; diced
- 3 carrots; peeled and diced
- 3 tbsps. of olive oil
- 1 tsp. of salt

Directions:

1. Add all Ingredients to a Crock Pot and stir well.
2. Cover and cook on low for 6 hours.
3. Purée the soup until smooth using an immersion blender.
4. Season soup with pepper and salt.

5. Serve and enjoy.

Nutrition:

- Calories 126
- Fat 5 g
- Carbohydrates 13 g
- Sugar 7 g
- Protein 5 g
- Cholesterol 0 mg

Mixed Vegetable Soup

Preparation time: 5 minutes

Cooking time: 30 minutes

Servings: 4

Ingredients:

- 1 tablespoon of olive oil
- 1 chopped leek
- 1 chopped bok choy
- 4 chopped carrots
- 2 cloves of minced garlic
- 1 chopped zucchini
- 2 chopped tomatoes
- 1 cup of garbanzo beans soaked in water overnight (drained)
- 5 chopped potatoes
- 8 cups of broth
- 1 teaspoon of basil
- ½ cup of amaranth

Directions:

1. Sauté the first four Ingredients, adding garlic in the last minute.
2. Add the rest of the Ingredients and simmer on the stove for 25 minutes.

Nutrition:

- Calories: 241
- Fat: 2 g
- Fiber: 16 g
- Carbs: 9 g
- Protein: 22 g

Coconut and Shrimp Bisque

Preparation time: 10 minutes

Cooking time: 15 minutes

Servings: 4

Ingredients:

- ¼ cup of red curry paste
- 2 tablespoons of water
- 1 tablespoon of extra-virgin olive oil
- 1 bunch of scallions; sliced
- 1-pound medium (21-30 count) of shrimp; peeled and deveined
- 1 cup of frozen peas
- 1 red bell pepper; diced
- 1 (14-ounce) can of full-fat coconut milk
- Kosher salt

Directions:

1. In a small bowl, whisk together the red curry paste and water. Set aside.

2. Select roast/sauté and set to med. Press start/stop to start. Allow to preheat for 3 minutes.
3. Add the oil and scallions. Cook for 2 minutes.
4. Add the shrimp, peas, and bell pepper. Stir well to mix. Stir in the red curry paste. Cook for 5 minutes, or until the peas are soft.
5. Stir in coconut milk and cook for more 5 minutes or until shrimp is cooked through and the bisque is thoroughly heated.
6. Season with salt and serve immediately.

Nutrition:

- Calories: 460
- Total Fat: 32 g
- Saturated Fat: 23 g
- Cholesterol: 223 mg
- Sodium: 902 mg
- Carbohydrates: 16 g
- Fiber: 5 g
- Protein: 29 g

Healthy Chicken Kale Soup

Preparation time: 10 minutes

Cooking time: 6 hours 15 minutes

Servings: 6

Ingredients:

- 2 lb. of chicken breasts; skinless and boneless
- 1/4 cup of fresh lemon juice
- 5 oz. of baby kale
- 32 oz. of chicken stock
- 1/2 cup of olive oil
- 1 large onion; sliced
- 14 oz. of chicken broth
- 1 tbsp. of extra-virgin olive oil
- Salt

Directions:

1. Heat the extra-virgin olive oil in a pan over medium heat.
2. Season chicken with salt and place in the hot pan.
3. Cover pan and cook chicken for 15 minutes.
4. Remove chicken from the pan and shred it using forks.

5. Add shredded chicken to a Crock Pot.
6. Add sliced onion, olive oil, and broth to a blender and blend until properly mixed.
7. Pour blended mixture into the Crock Pot.
8. Add the remaining Ingredients to the Crock Pot and stir well.
9. Cover and cook on low for 6 hours.
10. Stir well and serve.

Nutrition:

- Calories 493
- Fat 33 g
- Carbohydrates 8 g
- Sugar 9 g
- Protein 47 g
- Cholesterol 135 mg

Potato Soup

Preparation time: 5 minutes

Cooking time: 30 minutes

Servings: 4

Ingredients:

- 2 tablespoons of olive oil
- 1 diced onion
- 4 minced cloves of garlic
- 1 teaspoon of thyme
- 1 bay leaf
- 4 diced red potatoes
- 6 cups of water
- 1 sliced leek
- 3 diced celery stalks
- 2 teaspoons of salt
- ¼ teaspoon of pepper

Directions:

1. Sauté onion, garlic, thyme, and bay leaf in oil until translucent.

2. Add the rest of the Ingredients and simmer for about 20 minutes.

Nutrition:

- Calories: 267
- Fat: 13 g
- Fiber: 14 g
- Carbs: 17 g
- Protein: 10 g

Richard's Best Chicken

Preparation time: 5 minutes

Cooking time: 30 minutes

Servings: 4

Ingredients:

- 2 tablespoons of olive oil
- 8 chicken thighs
- 6 cloves of garlic
- 1 jar of artichoke hearts; drained
- ¾ cup of chicken broth
- 3 fresh squeezed oranges
- 1 sliced Meyer lemon
- ¼ cup of capers
- ½ cup of lives

Directions:

1. In a cast-iron skillet, fry chicken on all sides in oil until skin is golden and crispy. Remove from skillet.

2. Sauté garlic and artichokes for a couple of minutes, add chicken (skin up). Pour in the rest of the Ingredients and bring to a boil.
3. Place skillet with all Ingredients uncovered in a 3500 F oven for 30 minutes.

Nutrition:

- Calories: 285
- Fat: 28 g
- Fiber: 7 g
- Carbs: 34 g
- Protein: 23 g

Lamb Stew

Preparation time: 10 minutes

Cooking time: 8 hours

Servings: 2

Ingredients:

- 1/2 lb. of lean lamb; boneless and cubed
- 2 tbsps. of lemon juice
- 1/2 onion; chopped
- 2 garlic cloves; minced
- 2 fresh thyme sprigs
- 1/4 tsp. of turmeric
- 1/4 cup of green olives; sliced
- 1/2 tsp. of black pepper
- 1/4 tsp. of salt

Directions:

1. Add all the Ingredients into a crock pot and stir well.
2. Cover and cook on low for 8 hours.
3. Stir well and serve.

Nutrition:

- Calories 297
- Fat 20.3 g
- Carbohydrates 4 g
- Sugar 5 g
- Protein 21 g
- Cholesterol 80 mg

Goulash

Preparation time: 15 minutes

Cooking time: 55 minutes

Servings: 6

Ingredients:

- ½ cup all-purpose flour
- 1 tablespoon of kosher salt
- ½ teaspoon of freshly ground black pepper
- 2 pounds' of beef stew meat
- 2 tablespoons of canola oil
- 1 medium red bell pepper; seeded and chopped
- 4 garlic cloves; minced
- 1 large yellow onion; diced
- 2 tablespoons of smoked paprika
- 1½ pounds of small Yukon gold potatoes; halved
- 2 cups of beef broth
- 2 tablespoons of tomato paste
- ¼ cup of sour cream Fresh parsley, for garnish

Directions:

1. Select burn/sauté and set to start. Press start/stop to start. Allow to preheat for 5 minutes.
2. Mix together the flour, salt, and pepper in a small bowl. Dip the pieces of beef into the flour mixture, shaking off any extra flour.
3. Add the oil and allow to heat for 1 minute. Place the meat in the pot and brown it on all sides, for about 10 minutes.
4. Add the bell pepper, garlic, onion, and smoked paprika. Sauté for about 8 minutes or until the onion is translucent.
5. Add the potatoes, beef stock, and ingredient and stir.
6. Select pressure and set to low. Set time to 30 minutes. Select start/stop to start.
7. When the pressure cooking is finished, relieve the pressure by moving the pressure discharge valve to the vent position. Cautiously remove top unit where heat passes through while delivering pressure.
8. Add the soured cream and blend thoroughly. Garnish with parsley, if desired, and serve immediately.

Nutrition:

- Calories: 413
- Fat: 13 g
- Saturated fat: 4 g

- Cholesterol: 98 mg
- Sodium: 432 mg
- Carbohydrates: 64 g
- Fiber: 5 g
- Protein: 37 g

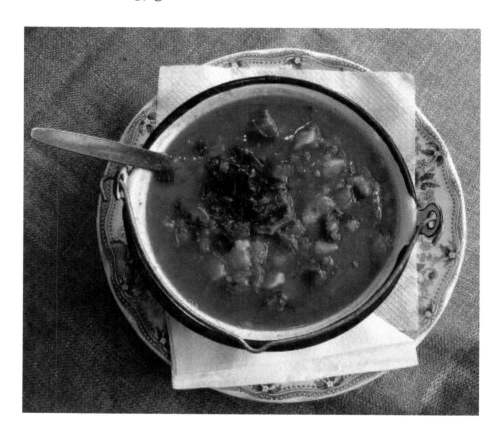

Loaded Potato Soup

Preparation time: 15 minutes

Cooking time: 30 minutes

Servings: 6

Ingredients:

- 5 slices of bacon; chopped
- 1 onion; chopped
- 3 garlic cloves; minced
- 4 pounds of russet potatoes; peeled and chopped
- 4 cups of chicken broth
- 1 cup of whole milk
- ½ teaspoon of sea salt
- ½ teaspoon of freshly ground black pepper
- 1½ cups of shredded cheddar cheese
- Sour cream; for serving (optional)
- Chopped fresh chives; for serving (optional)

Directions:

1. Add the bacon, onion, and garlic. Cook for 5 minutes, stirring occasionally. Put aside some of the bacon for garnish.

2. Add the potatoes and chicken stock. Setup pressure lid, making sure the pressure release valve is in the seal position.

3. Select pressure and set to high. Set time to 10 minutes, then press start/stop to start.

4. At the point when pressure cooking is finished, fast relieve the pressure by moving the pressure discharge valve to the vent position. Cautiously remove top unit where heat passes through while delivering pressure.

5. Add the milk and mash the Ingredients until the soup reaches your required consistency. Season with the salt and black pepper. Sprinkle the cheese evenly over the top of the soup. Close crisping lid.

6. Select broil and set time to 5 minutes. Press start/stop to start.

7. When cooking is complete, top with the reserved crispy bacon and serve with soured cream and chives (if using).

Nutrition:

- Calories: 468
- Total fat: 19 g

- Saturated fat: 9 g
- Cholesterol: 51 mg
- Sodium: 1041 mg
- Carbohydrates: 53 g
- Fiber: 8 g
- Protein: 23 g

Butternut Squash, Apple, Bacon and Orzo Soup

Preparation time: 10 minutes

Cooking time: 28 minutes

Servings: 8

Ingredients:

- 4 slices of uncooked bacon; cut into ½-inch pieces
- 12 ounces of butternut squash; peeled and cubed
- 1 green apple; cut into small cubes
- Kosher salt
- Freshly ground black pepper
- 1 tablespoon of minced fresh oregano
- 2 quarts (64 ounces) of chicken stock
- 1 cup of orzo

Directions:

1. Select roast/sauté and set temperature to high. Press start/stop to start. Allow to preheat for 5 minutes.

2. Place the bacon in the pot and cook, stirring frequently, for about 5 minutes, or until fat is produced and the bacon starts to brown. Using a slotted spoon, transfer the bacon to a paper towel-lined plate to drain, leaving the rendered bacon fat in the pot.

3. Add the butternut squash, apple, salt, pepper, and sauté until partially soft, or for about 5 minutes. Stir in the oregano.

4. Add the bacon back to the pot alongside the chicken broth. Bring to a boil for about 10 minutes, then add the orzo. Cook for about 8 minutes, or until the orzo is soft. Serve.

Nutrition:

- Calories: 247
- Total Fat: 7 g
- Saturated Fat: 2 g
- Cholesterol: 17 mg
- Sodium: 563 mg
- Carbohydrates: 33 g
- Fiber: 3 g
- Protein: 12 g

Delicious Chicken Soup

Preparation time: 10 minutes

Cooking time: 4 hours 30 minutes

Servings: 4

Ingredients:

- 1 lb. of chicken breasts; boneless and skinless
- 2 tbsp. of fresh basil; chopped
- 1 1/2 cups of mozzarella cheese; shredded
- 2 garlic cloves; minced
- 1 tbsp. of Parmesan cheese; grated
- 2 tbsp. of dried basil
- 2 cups of chicken stock
- 28 oz. of tomatoes; diced
- 1/4 tsp. of pepper
- 1/2 tsp. of salt

Directions:

1. Add chicken, Parmesan cheese, dried basil, tomatoes, garlic, pepper, and salt to a Crock Pot and stir well to mix.
2. Cover and cook on low for 4 hours.

3. Add fresh basil and mozzarella cheese and stir well.
4. Cover again and cook for 30 more minutes or until cheese is melted.
5. Remove chicken from the Crock Pot and shred using fork.
6. Return shredded chicken to the Crock Pot and stir to mix.
7. Serve and enjoy.

Nutrition:

- Calories: 299
- Fat: 16 g
- Carbohydrates: 3 g
- Sugar: 6 g
- Protein: 38 g
- Cholesterol: 108 mg

Spicy Chicken Pepper Stew

Preparation time: 10 minutes

Cooking time: 6 hours

Servings: 6

Ingredients:

- 3 chicken breasts; skinless and boneless, cut into small pieces
- 1 tsp. of garlic; minced
- 1 tsp. of ground ginger
- 2 tsp. of olive oil
- 2 tsp. of soy sauce
- 1 tbsp. of fresh lemon juice
- 1/2 cup of green onions; sliced
- 1 tbsp. of crushed red pepper
- 8 oz. of chicken stock
- 1 bell pepper; chopped
- 1 green chili pepper; sliced
- 2 jalapeño peppers; sliced
- 1/2 tsp. of black pepper
- 1/4 tsp. of sea salt

Directions:

1. Add all Ingredients to a large bowl and blend well. Place in the refrigerator overnight.
2. Pour marinated chicken mixture into a Crock Pot.
3. Cover and cook on low for 6 hours.
4. Stir well and serve.

Nutrition:

- Calories: 171
- Fat: 4 g
- Carbohydrates: 7 g
- Sugar: 7 g
- Protein: 22 g
- Cholesterol: 65 mg

Beef Chili

Preparation time: 10 minutes

Cooking time: 8 hours

Servings: 6

Ingredients:

- 1 lb. of ground beef
- 1 tsp. of garlic powder
- 1 tsp. of paprika
- 3 tsp. of chili powder
- 1 tbsp. of Worcestershire sauce
- 1 tbsp. of fresh parsley; chopped
- 1 tsp. of onion powder
- 25 oz. of tomatoes; chopped
- 4 carrots; chopped
- 1 onion; diced
- 1 bell pepper; diced
- 1/2 tsp. of sea salt

Directions:

1. Brown the ground meat in a pan over high heat until meat is no longer pink.
2. Transfer meat to a Crock Pot.
3. Add bell pepper, tomatoes, carrots, and onion to the Crock Pot and stir well.
4. Add the remaining Ingredients and stir well.
5. Cover and cook on low for 8 hours.
6. Serve and enjoy.

Nutrition:

- Calories: 152
- Fat: 4 g
- Carbohydrates: 4 g
- Sugar: 8 g
- Protein: 18 g
- Cholesterol 51 mg

Healthy Spinach Soup

Preparation time: 10 minutes

Cooking time: 3 hours

Servings: 8

Ingredients:

- 3 cups of frozen spinach; chopped, thawed, and drained
- 8 oz. of cheddar cheese; shredded
- 1 egg; lightly beaten
- 10 oz. of can cream chicken soup
- 8 oz. of cream cheese; softened

Directions:

1. Add spinach to a large bowl. Purée the spinach.
2. Add egg, chicken soup, cheese, and pepper to the spinach purée and blend well.
3. Transfer spinach mixture to a Crock Pot.
4. Cover and cook on low for 3 hours.
5. Stir in cheddar and serve.

Nutrition:

- Calories: 256
- Fat: 29 g
- Carbohydrates: 1 g
- Sugar: 0.5 g
- Protein: 11 g
- Cholesterol: 84 mg

Mexican Chicken Soup

Preparation time: 10 minutes

Cooking time: 4 hours

Servings: 6

Ingredients:

- 1 1/2 lb. of chicken thighs, skinless and boneless
- 14 oz. of chicken stock
- 14 oz. of salsa
- 8 oz. of Monterey Jack cheese, shredded

Directions:

1. Place chicken into a Crock Pot.
2. Pour the remaining Ingredients over the chicken.
3. Cover and cook on high for 4 hours.
4. Remove chicken from Crock Pot and shred using a fork.
5. Return shredded chicken to the Crock Pot and stir well.
6. Serve and enjoy.

Nutrition:

- Calories: 371
- Fat: 15 g
- Carbohydrates: 7 g
- Sugar: 2 g
- Protein: 41 g
- Cholesterol: 135 mg

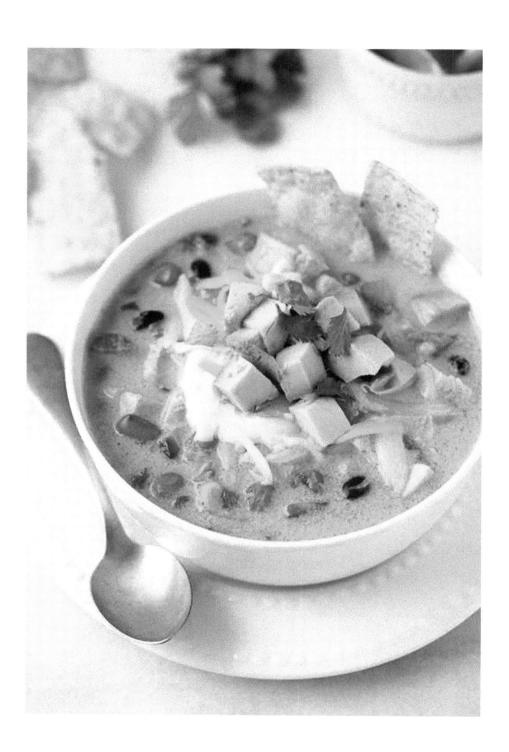

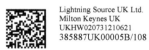

Lightning Source UK Ltd.
Milton Keynes UK
UKHW020731210621
385887UK00005B/108

9 781802 778717